rainbow bellies

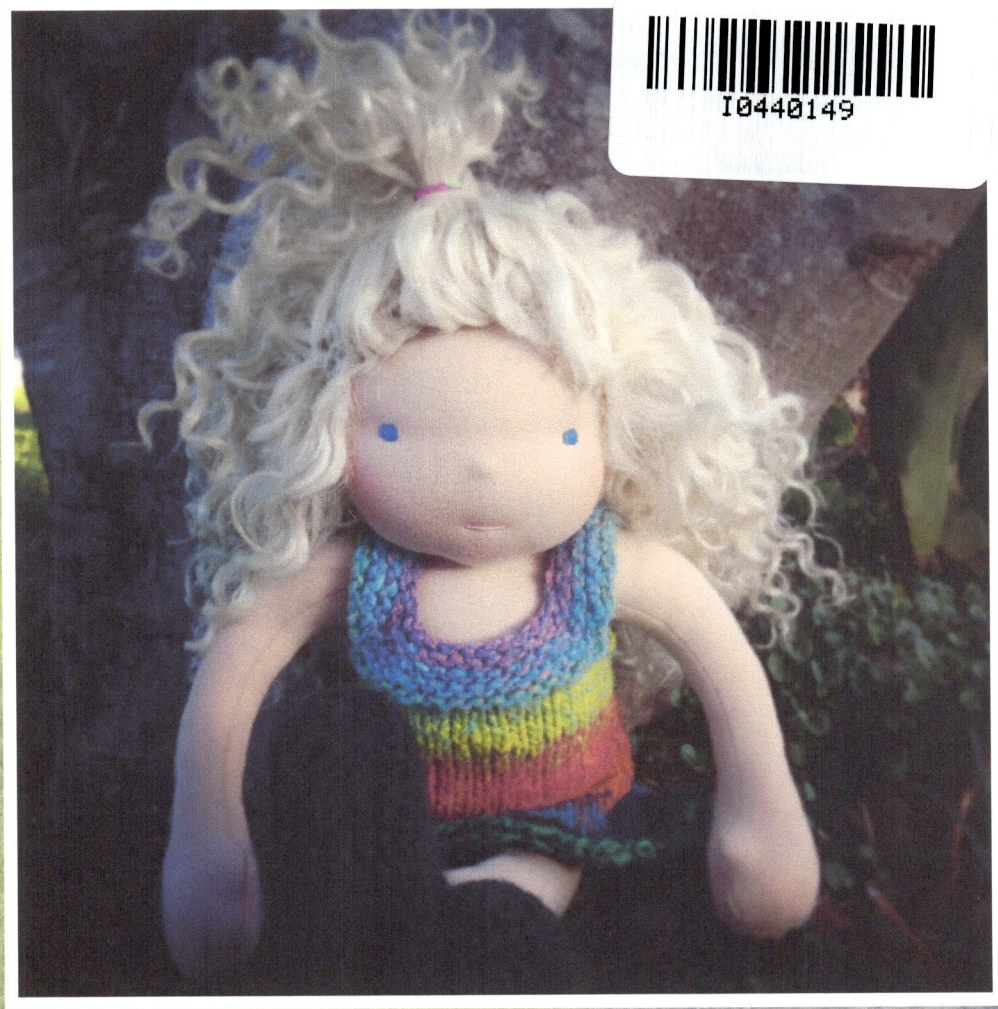

A Story to Help Children Cope with Food Sensitivities and Intolerances

Written and Illustrated by Nadine Thomson

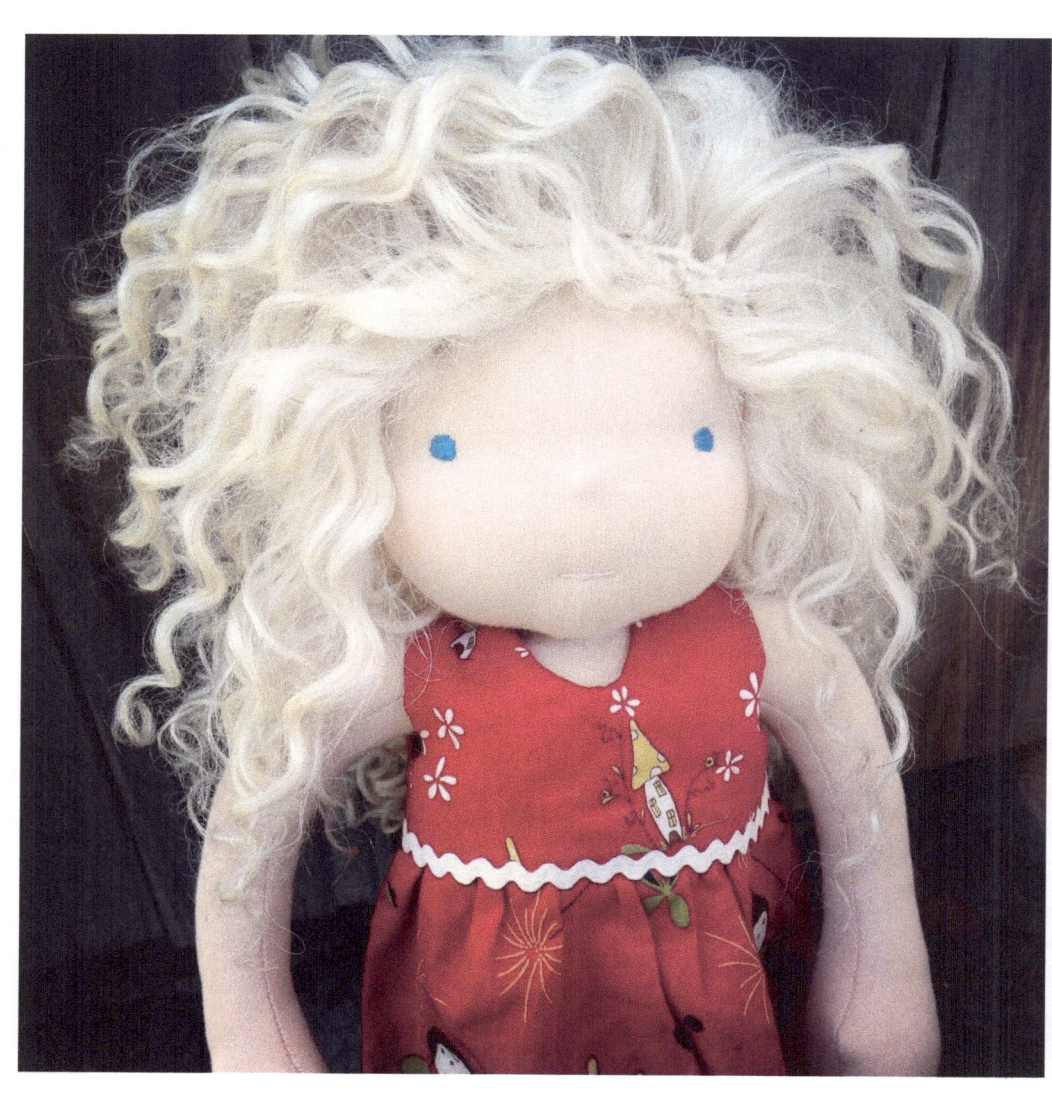

There once was a girl named Kaia Rose. She could be fun, happy and full of energy. She could also be cranky, tired and whingy!

Kaia Rose didn't like feeling upset, but something inside her made her feel that way.

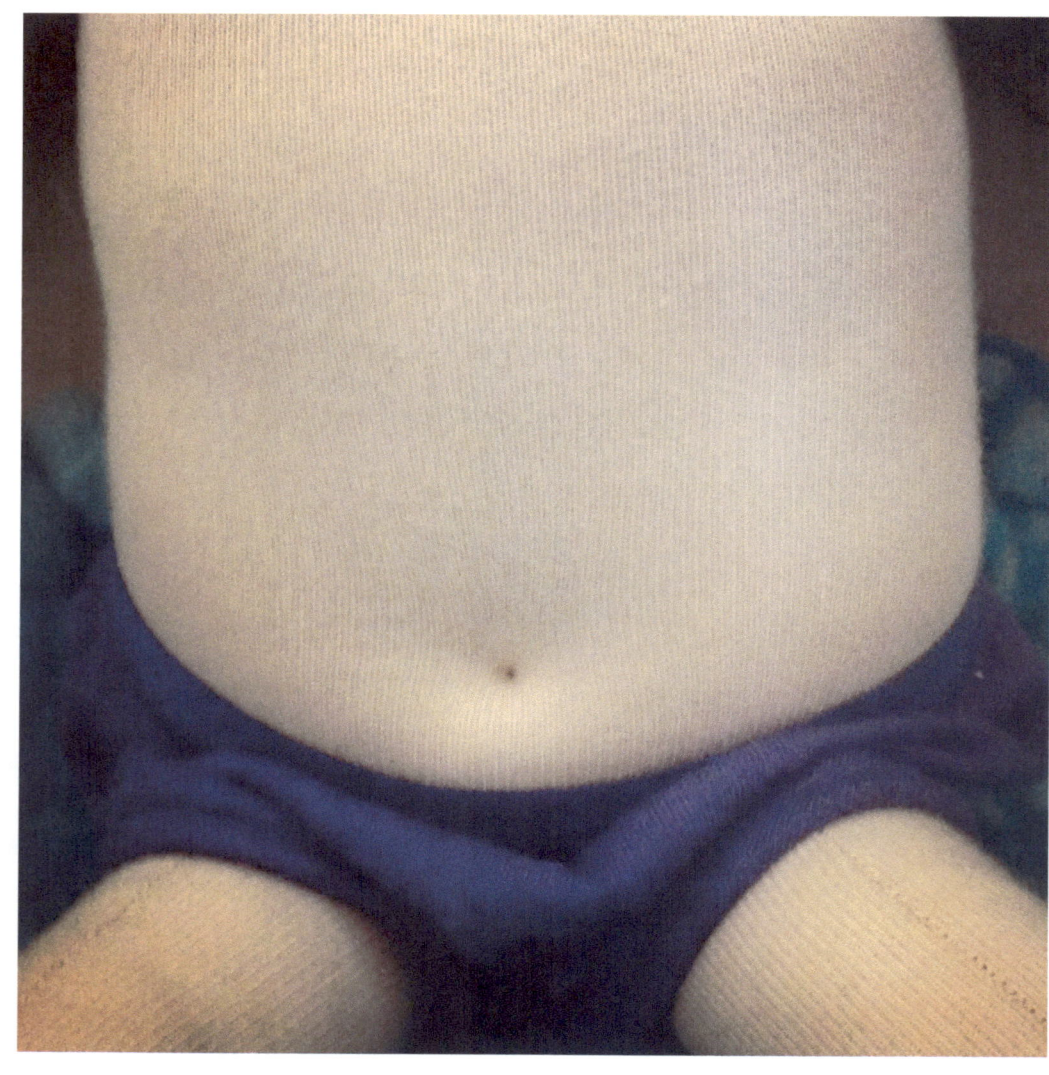

What was it that made her feel cranky, tired and whingy? Well, you see, it was her belly. Kaia Rose didn't know it yet, but her belly was sad.

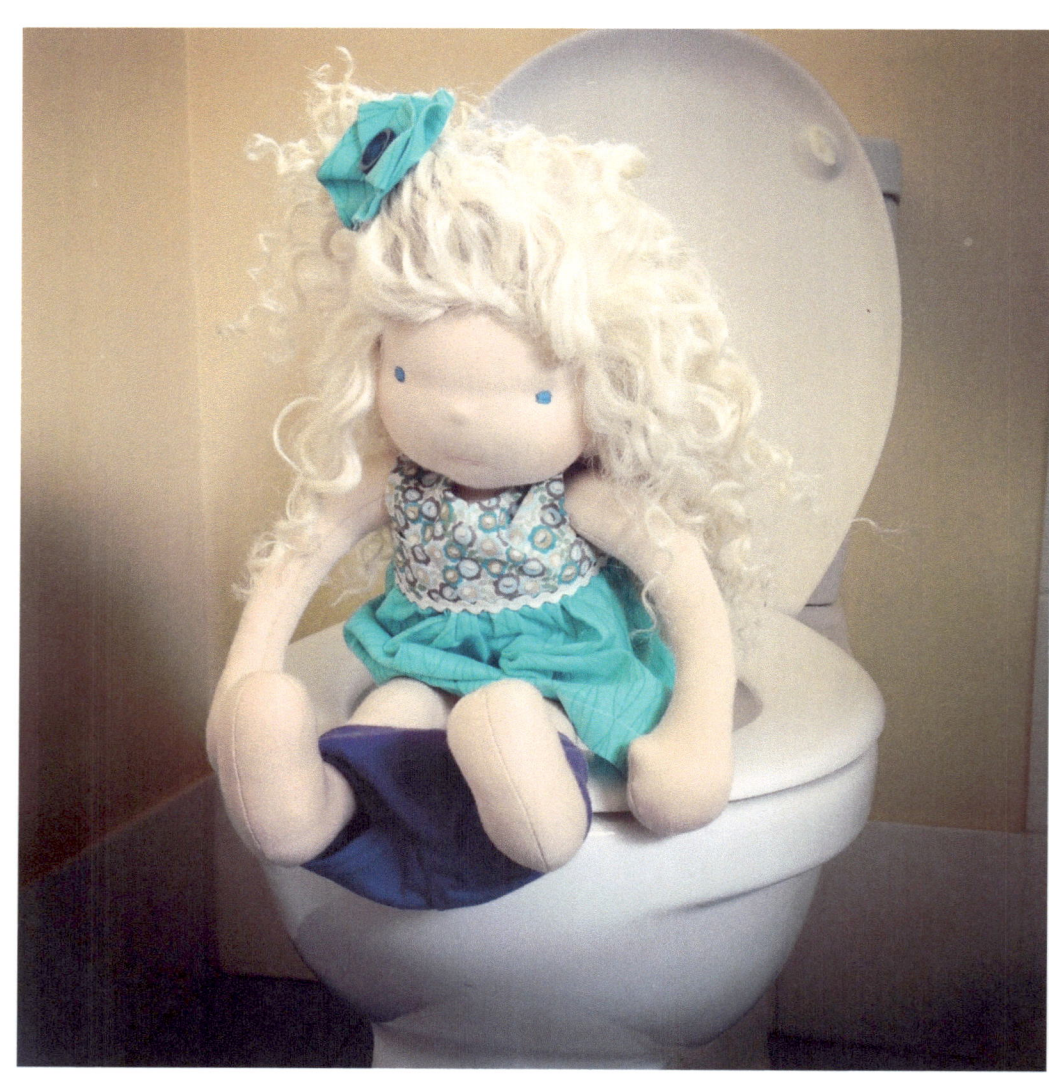

One day Kaia Rose was sitting on the toilet when she heard something. It wasn't a usual toilet sound, it sounded like a whisper. Kaia Rose listened hard and heard it again. It said, "help me." She realised that the whisper came from her belly.

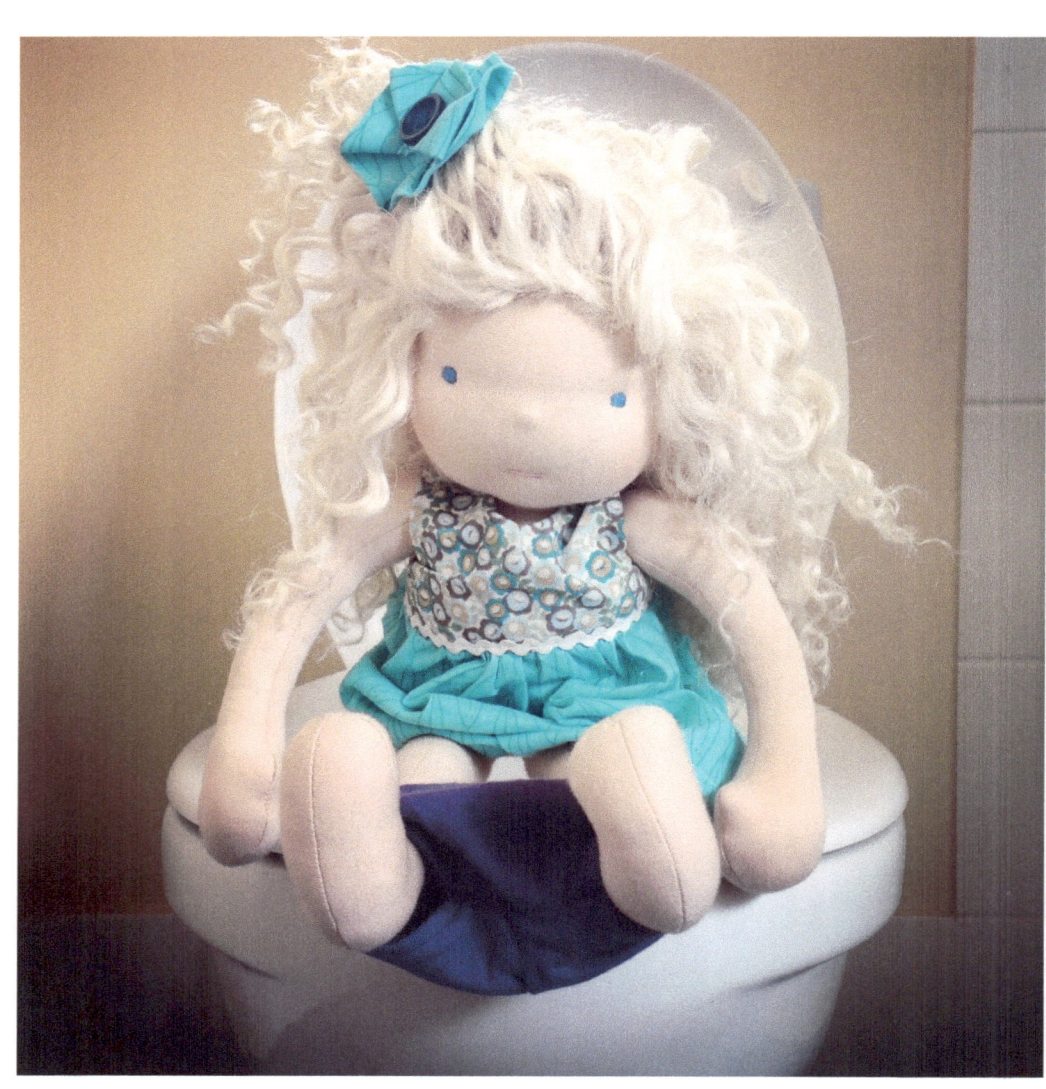

"How can I help you belly?" Kaia Rose asked.

"I'm running out of rainbows," it answered. "Rainbows make me happy."

"Rainbows?" she said. "I love rainbows too, but how can I get rainbows into my belly?"

"You can eat Rainbow Food," answered her belly, and it said no more.

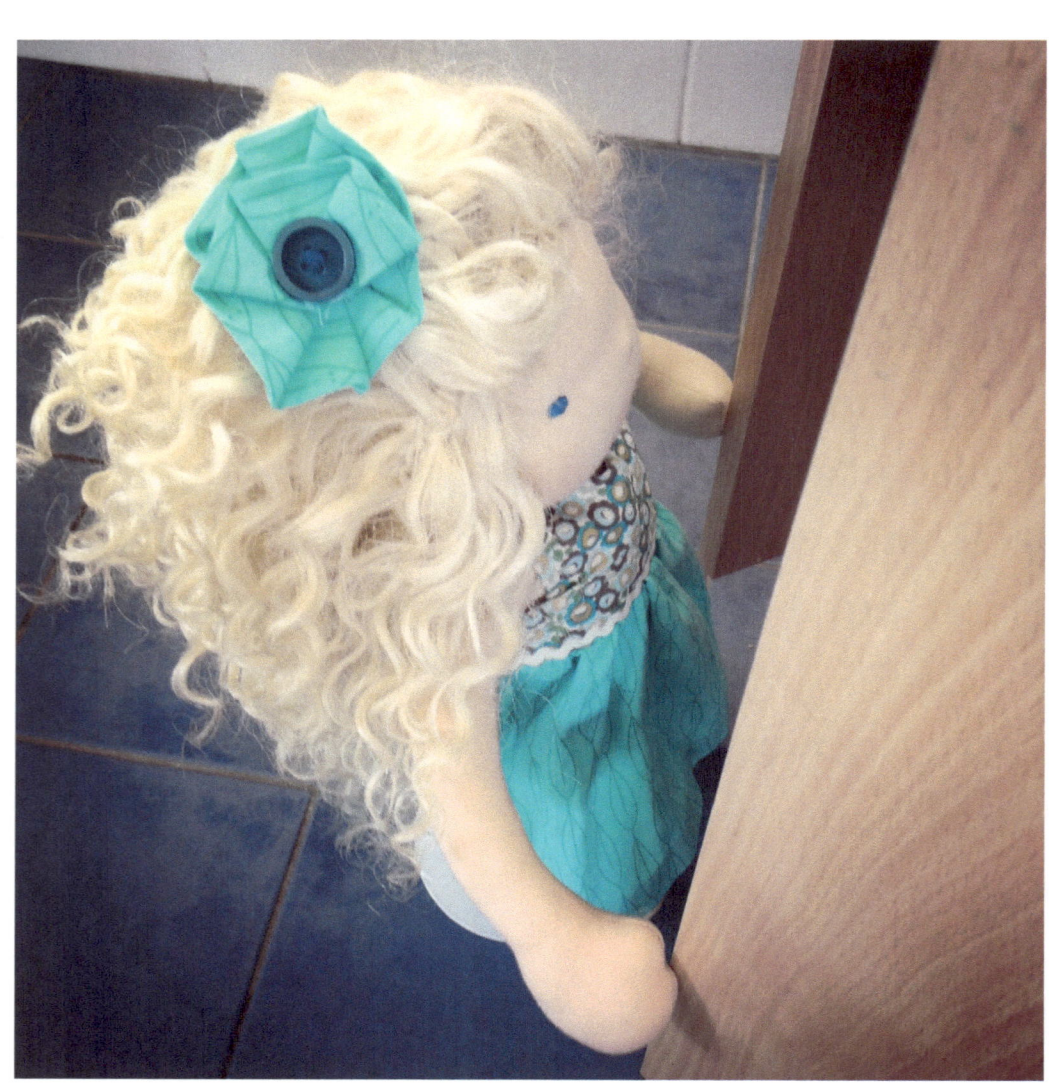

Kaia Rose wiped her bum, flushed the toilet and washed her hands. She sped off to the kitchen to look for rainbow food. She hunted high and low through the fridge and pantry looking for foods that she thought could be rainbowy. She loved rainbows, so she looked for all of her favourite foods.

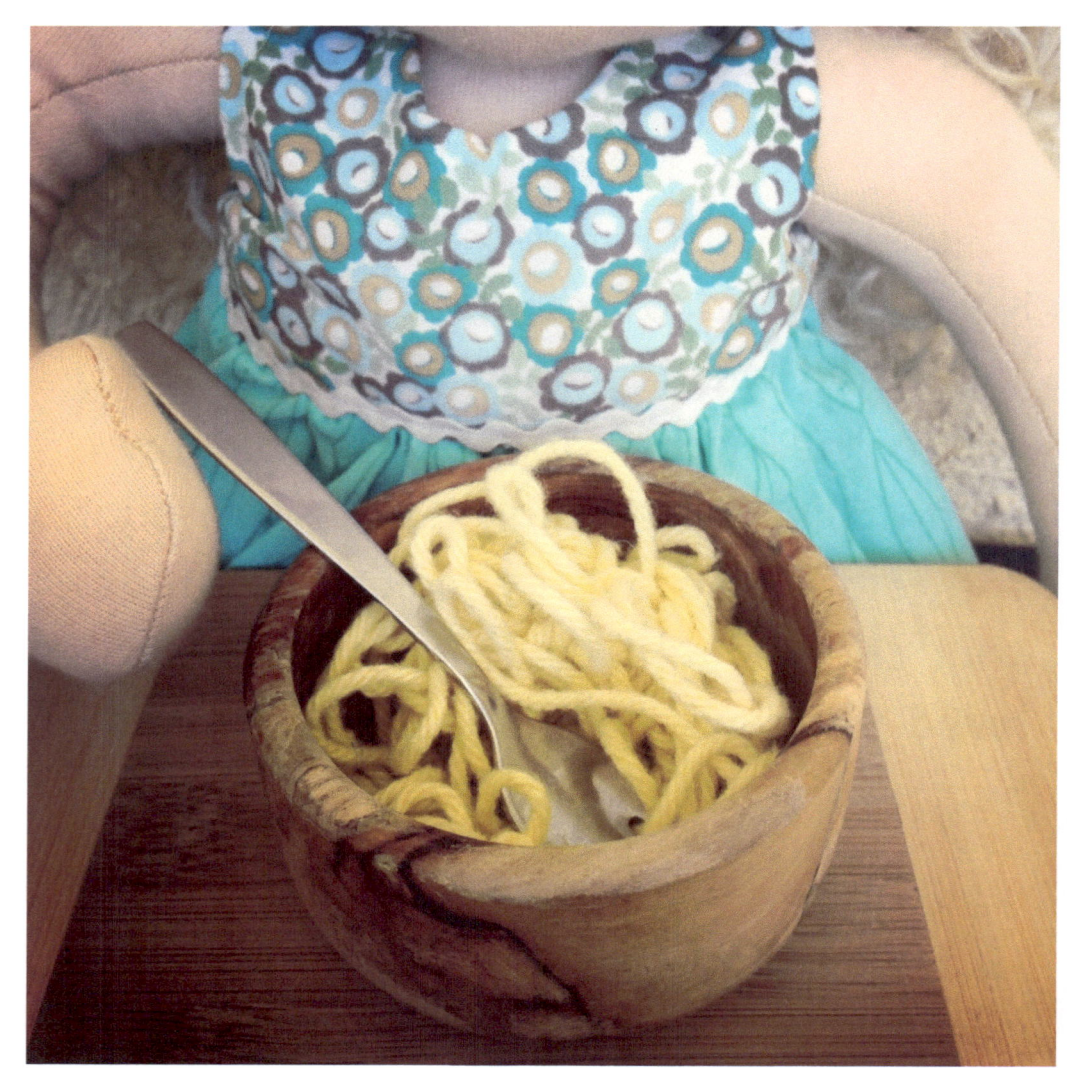

Kaia Rose loved pasta, so the first thing she thought she might try was a big bowl of Spaghetti.

After a few bites, her belly said, "GRUMBLE!"

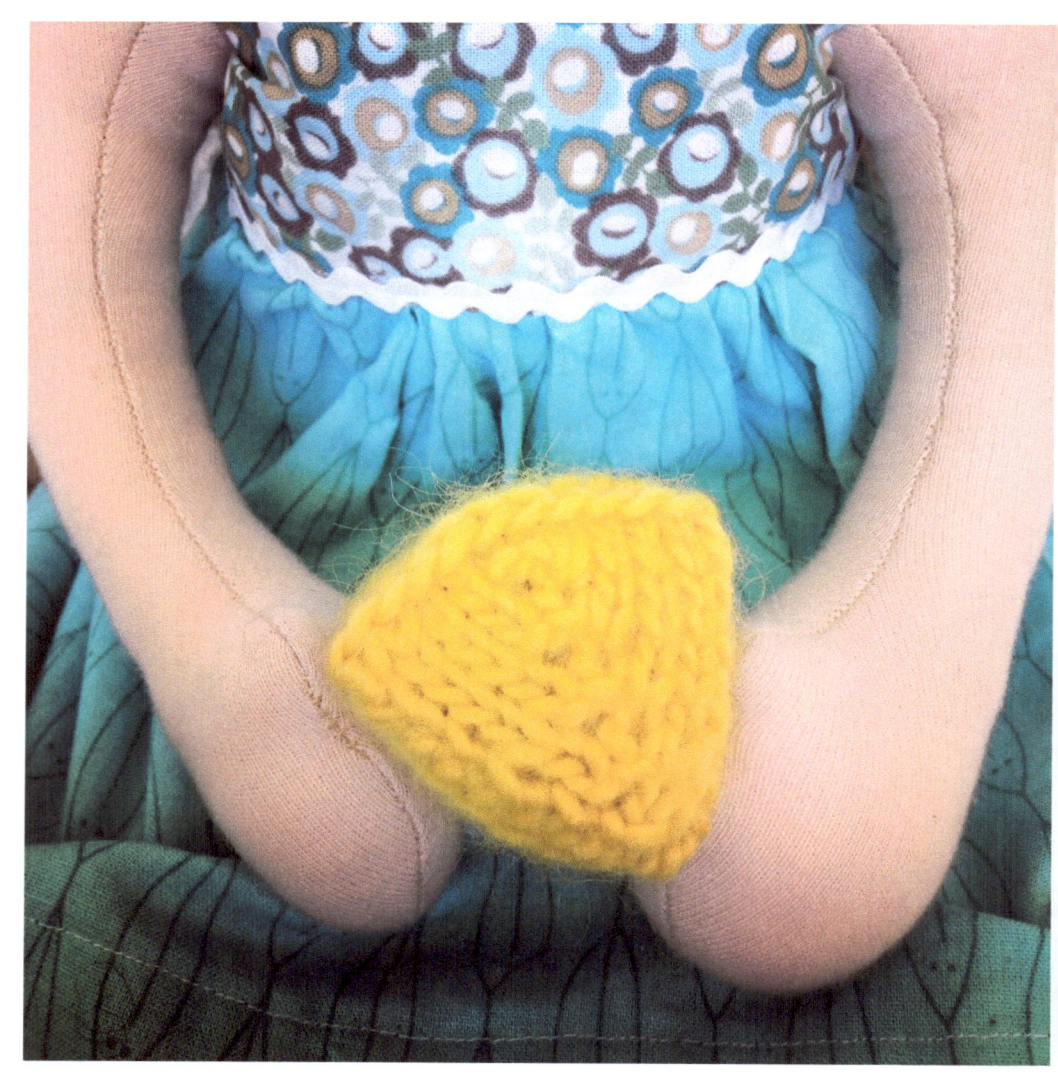

"Hmmm," she thought, "that didn't sound good. Well, I also love cheese, maybe this will give my belly some rainbows."

After a few bites, her belly said "GRUMBLE, GROAN!"

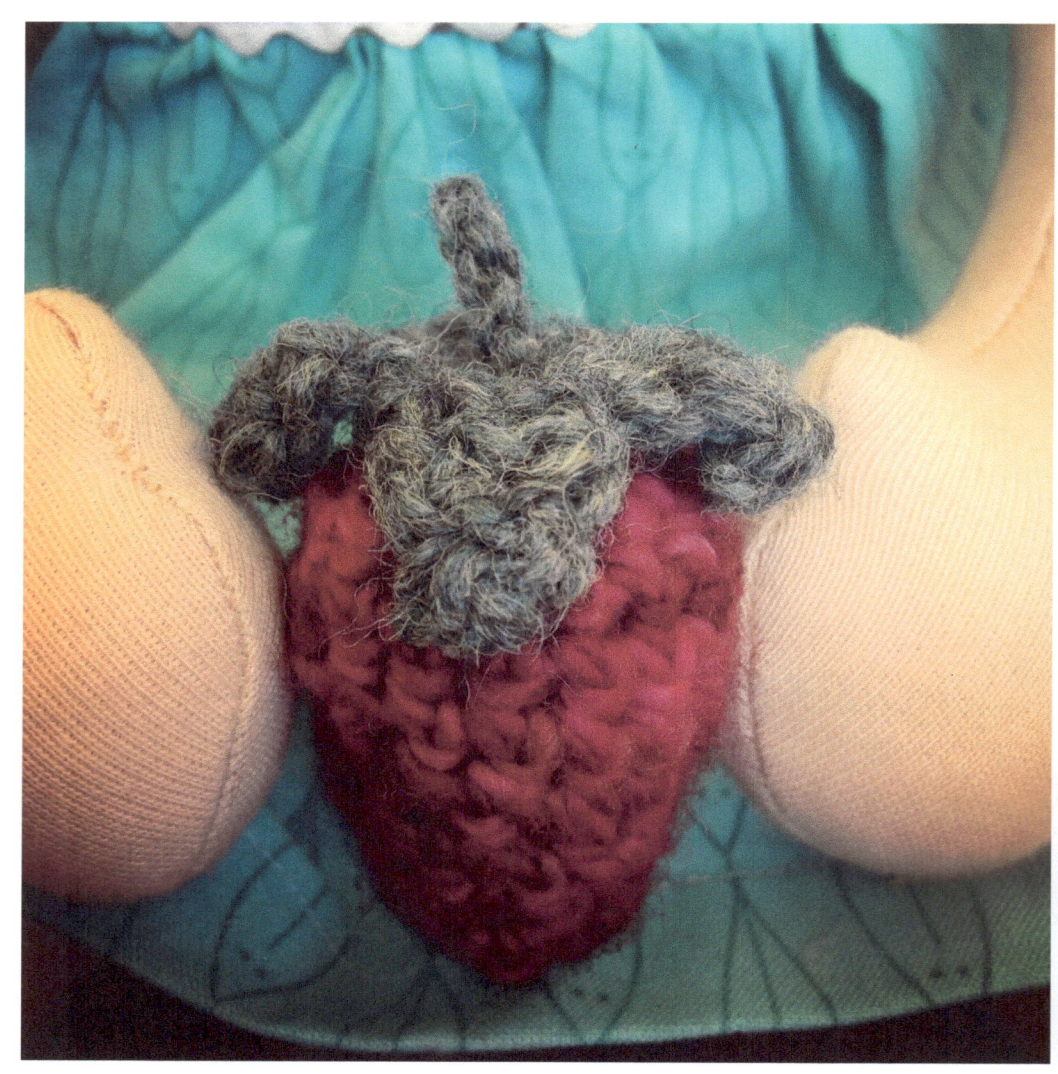

"Oh my," she thought. "Well, surely a juicy, ripe strawberry will make my belly happy!"

After a few bites, her belly said, "GRUMBLE, GROAN, SQUEAK!"

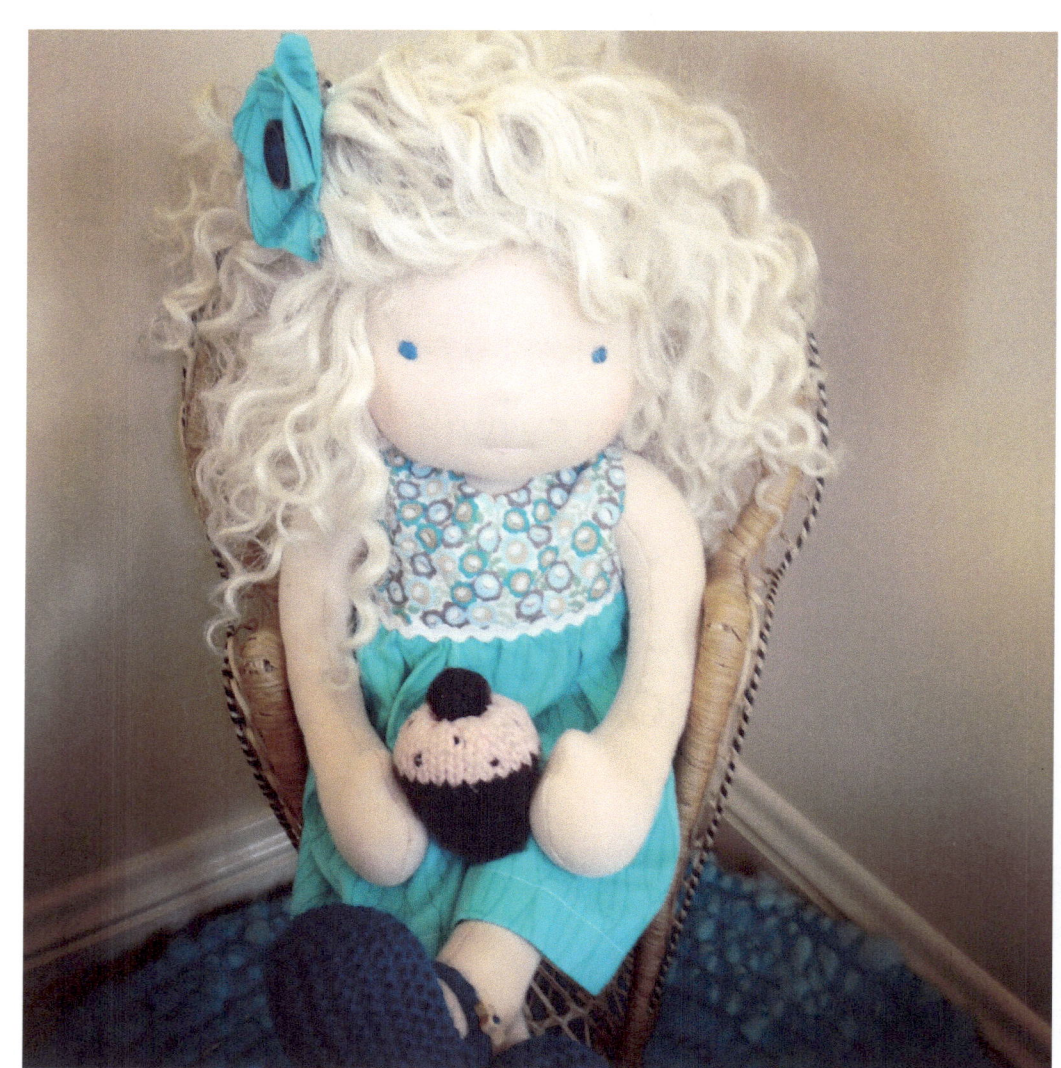

"Oh dear," Kaia Rose thought, "this is going to be trickier than I thought. None of these foods seem to make my belly happy." Just then she remembered her most favourite food in the whole entire world: cupcakes! She ran back to the kitchen, grabbed a cupcake then went to eat it in her favourite chair.

After a few bites her belly said "GRUMBLE, GROAN, SQUEAK, TOOT!"

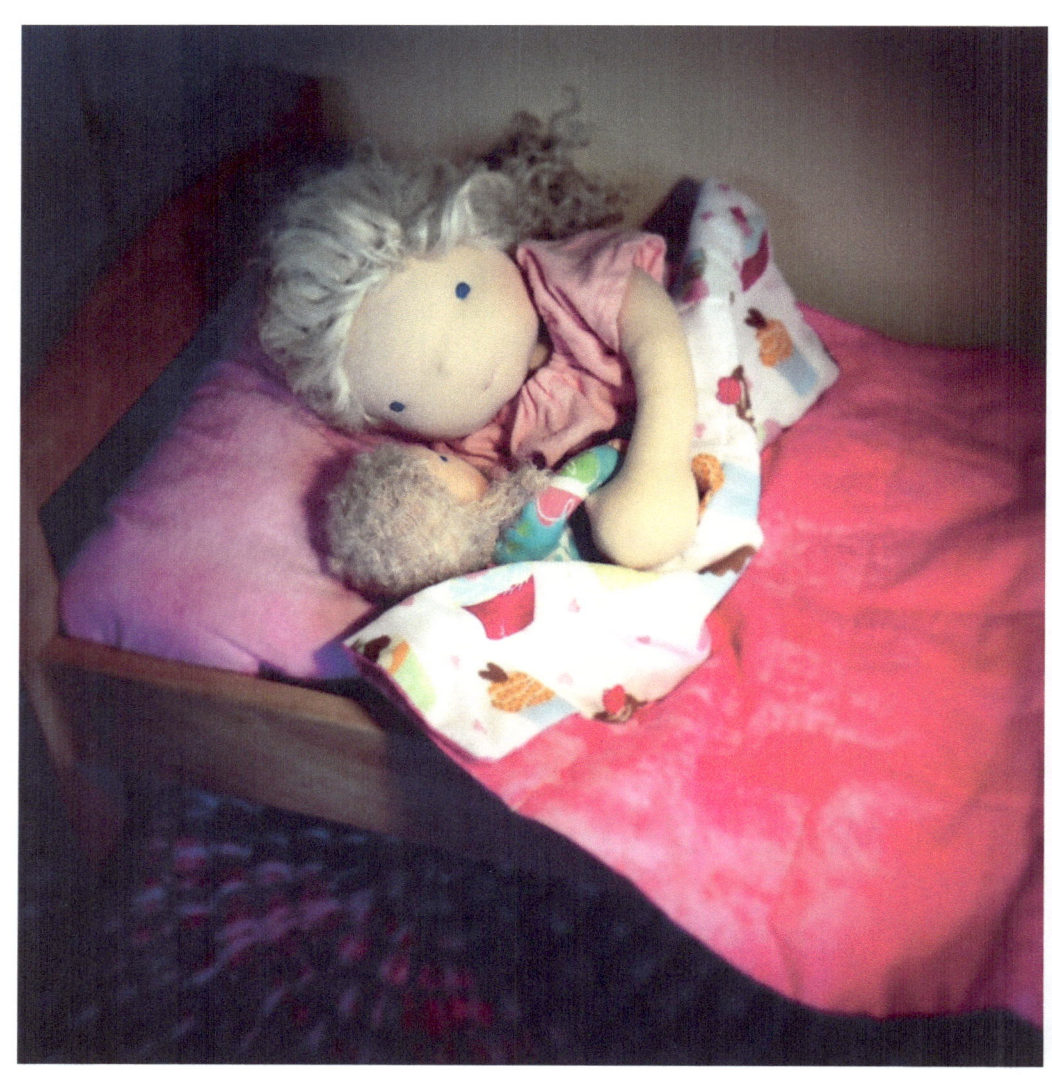

At bedtime Kaia Rose was feeling very discouraged and told her dolly Molly all about it. She held Molly extra tight that night. As she drifted off to sleep, she thought she heard another whisper. This time it said, "Find me some rainbows."

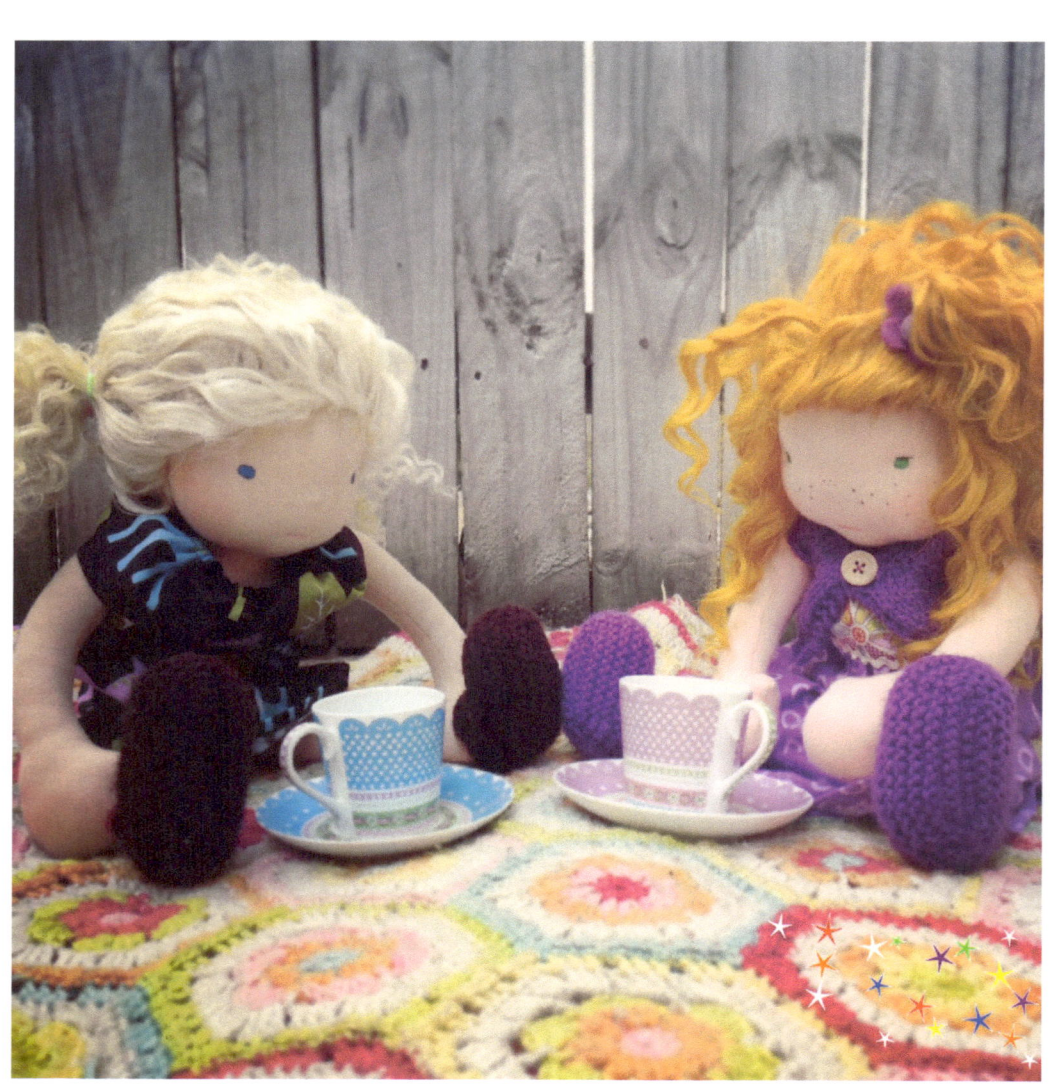

That night Kaia Rose had a dream. She dreamt she was having a tea party with her friend Hannah in the backyard. Suddenly, she spotted a shimmer of rainbow sparkles. Kaia Rose followed the sparkles and they led her to a huge beautiful garden, full of veggies and fruits of every colour of the rainbow. The sparkles faded and there appeared Mother Earth.

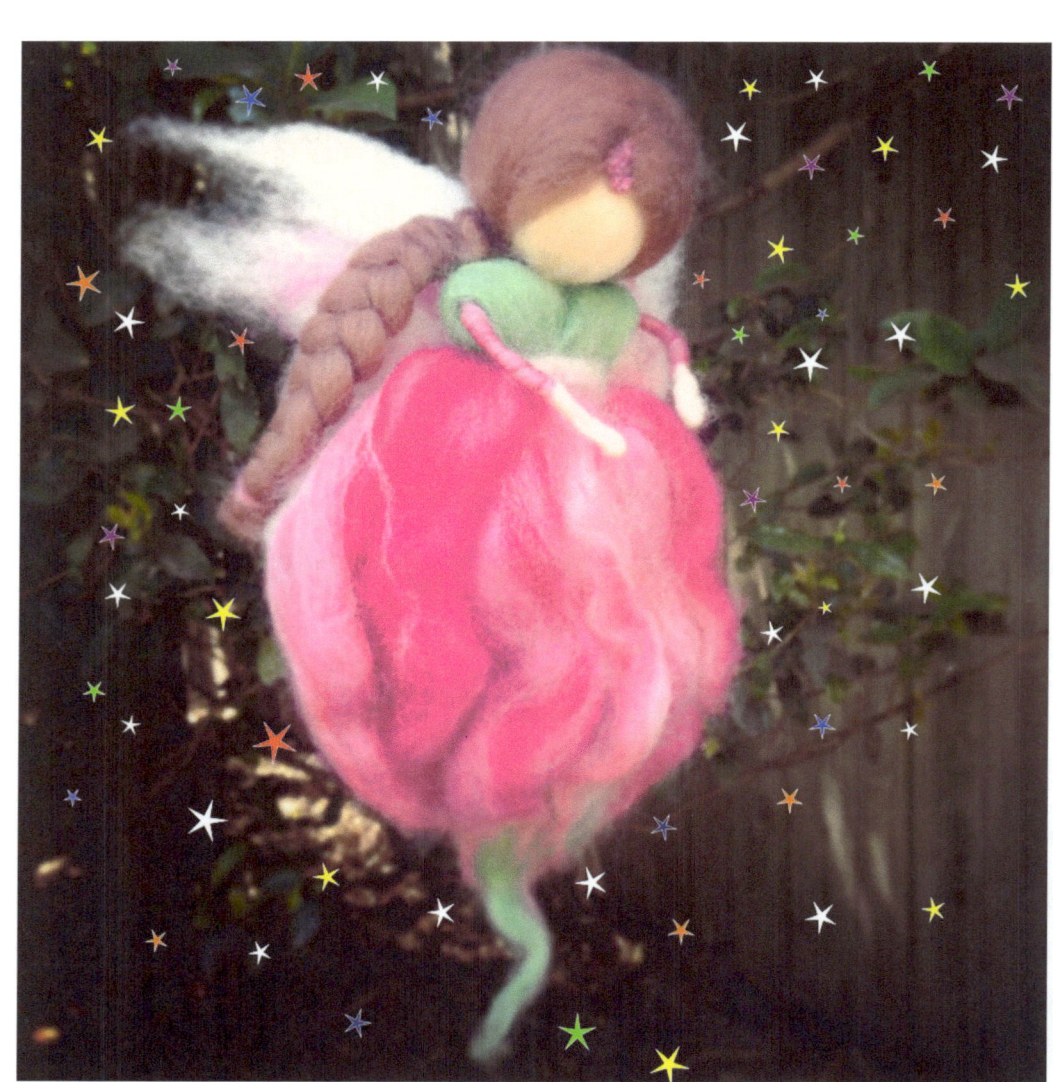

Mother Earth said to her:

"If you are looking for your rainbows
I will show you where they grow.
I, along with Father Sun,
Grow rainbow food for everyone.
Each child's belly likes a different colour
Your belly's favourite you must discover."

Then she disappeared into a shimmer of
rainbow sparkles.

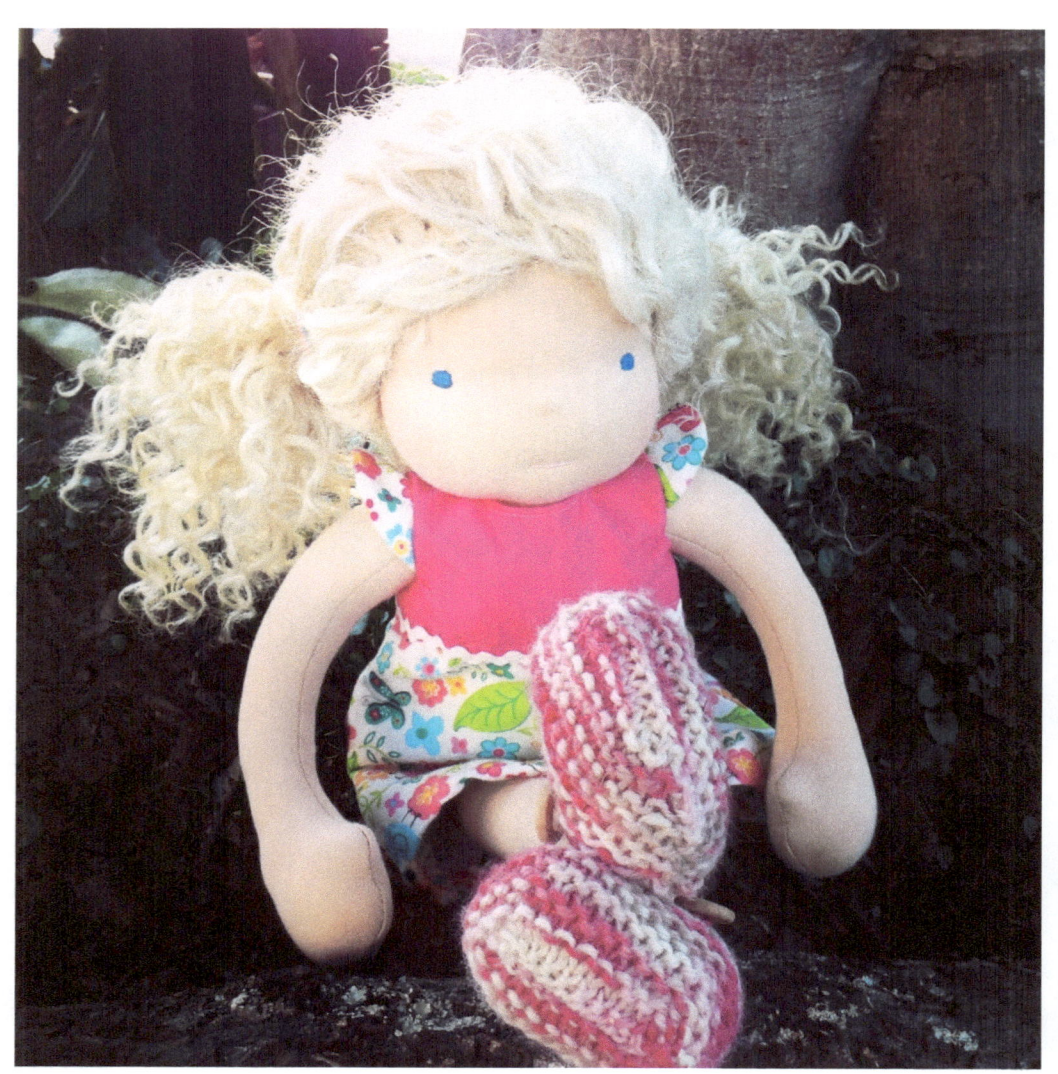

The next morning Kaia Rose woke up feeling happy and excited to find her very own rainbow foods.

Later that afternoon her Mum called her to help prepare dinner. Kaia Rose liked helping her Mum in the kitchen. They were making one of her favourites, chicken soup.

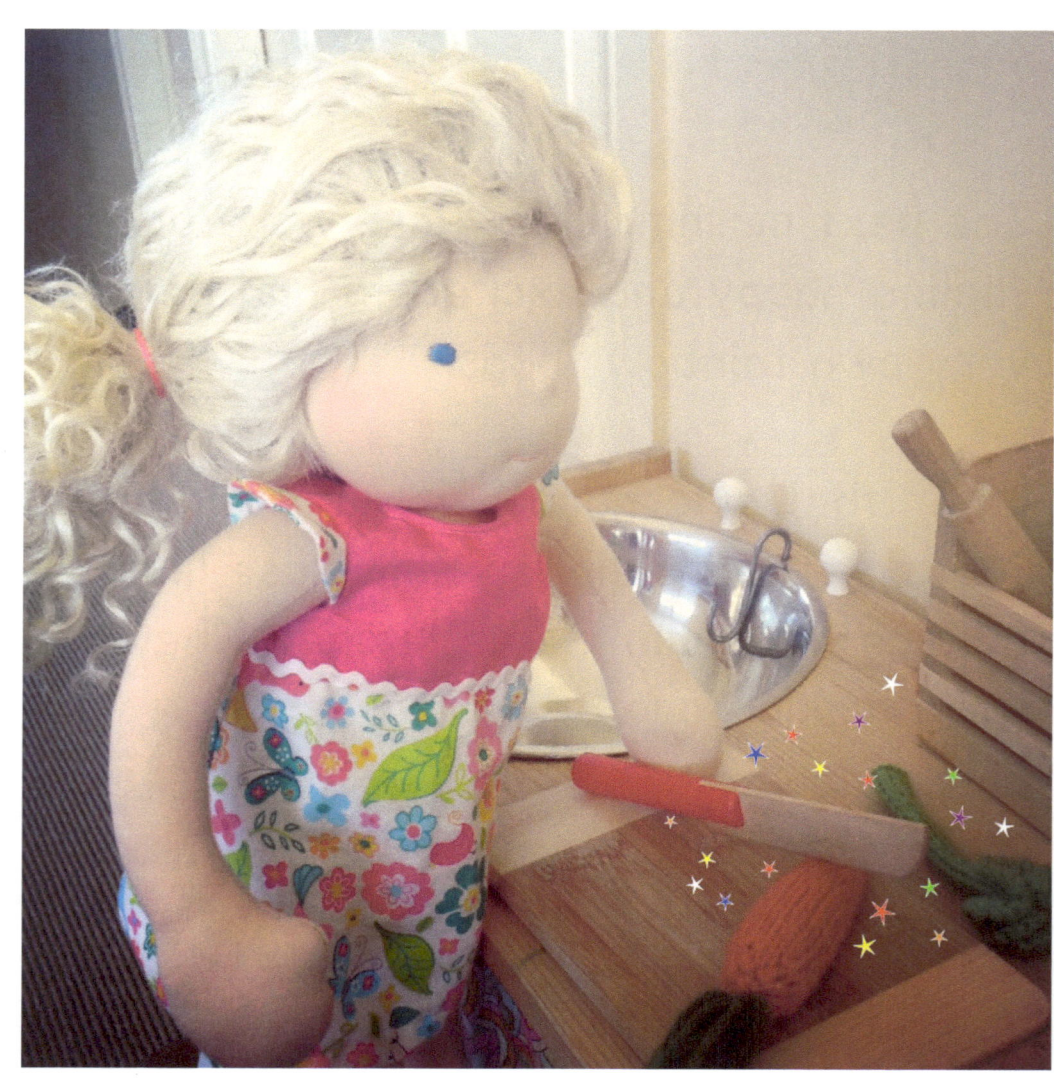

As Kaia Rose chopped the veggies, she thought she spotted some rainbow sparkles. A big smile spread across her face. Had she finally found some of her rainbow food?

After eating her chicken soup she, and her belly, felt happy. Her belly didn't grumble, groan, squeak or toot! She realised that finding her rainbow foods wasn't going to be so tricky after all.

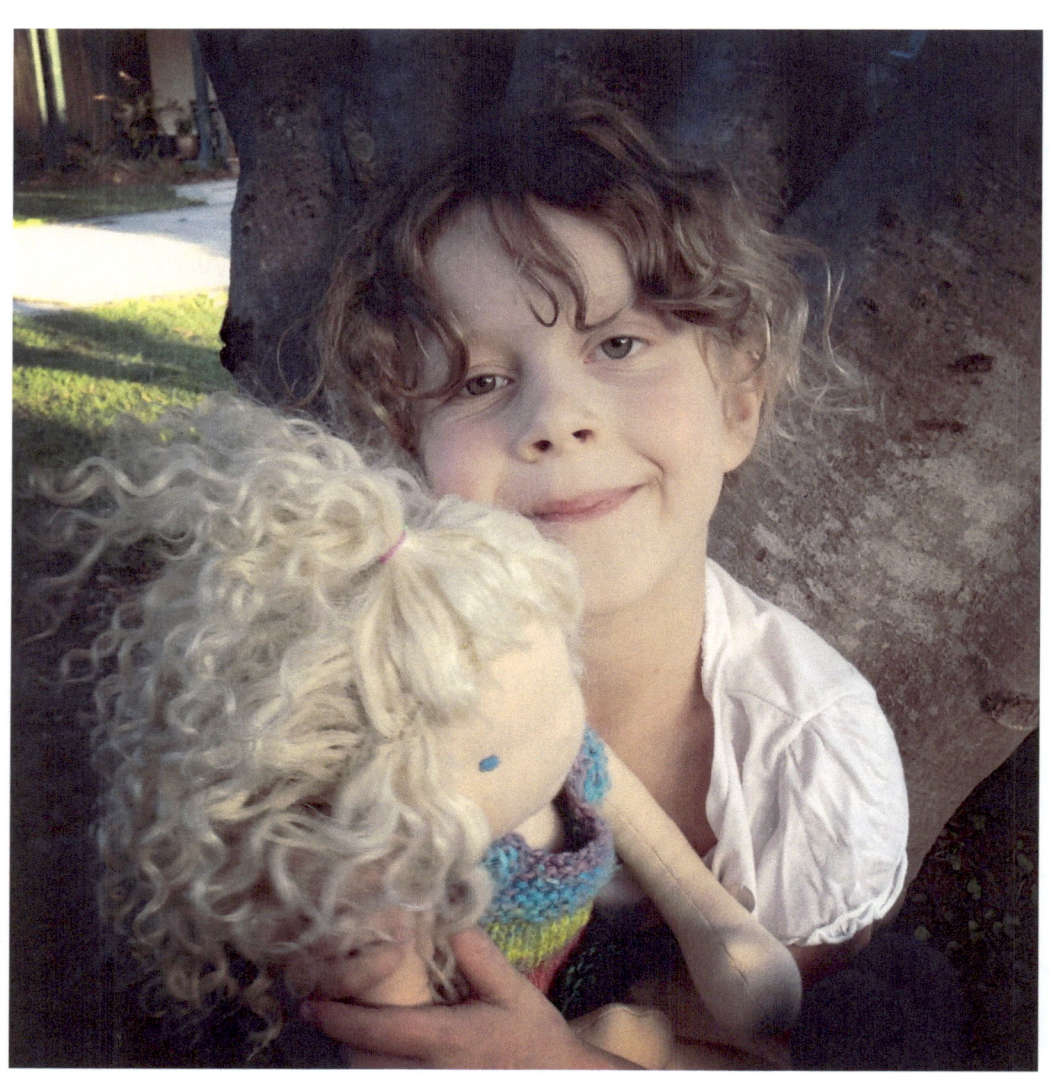

It took a long time, but Kaia Rose finally found all the foods that made her belly happy. She could still have plenty of her old favourites and discovered yummy new treats too (including delicious cupcakes made with her own rainbow ingredients!).

How about you? Have you found your rainbow foods?

Find them and you too can shine like a rainbow!

A Note from the Author:

This book was inspired by my daughter's battle with leaky gut. At 18 months she developed an itchy skin rash and suffered occasional diarrhoea and belly aches. Helping her has been a long, difficult journey. We tried many natural options; Homeopathy, Naturopathy, Kinesiology and food allergy tests (avoiding steroid cream at all costs). Determining a food intolerance is tricky, to say the least. We have been healing and sealing her gut with probiotics and trigger food avoidance and are finally seeing progress.

Having food intolerances is not only physically difficult for a child, but also emotionally. We heard a lot of "it's not fair" and "why can't I eat that" and attending a Birthday Party was a nightmare.

I believe in the healing power of stories. Children learn through stories, which bring complex concepts into the imaginary realm, where the child lives. This story has helped our little Kaia Rose and I hope it will help bring comfort to your little one too.

The dolls in this story are Waldorf Inspired. Their neutral facial expression help a child's imagination flourish. They can be happy, sad, angry, or frustrated, becoming a sympathetic companion on a child's journey. They are made with all natural materials, including wool, cotton, mohair, and LOVE!

For more information on our story and how to get your own custom made doll, please visit www.woolyroodolls.com

*All dolls and handmade items in this book were created by Wooly Roo Dolls (me) and all paintings by my daughters Kaia Rose and Lennox Elizabeth

xox Nadine

p.s Download your free audio version of this story at: http://www.woolyroodolls.com/rainbowbellies

www.ingramcontent.com/pod-product-compliance
Lightning Source LLC
Chambersburg PA
CBHW050918290526
45792CB00002B/807